Chicken Soup for the Soul®
Healthy Living:
Asthma

Chicken Soup for the Soul® Healthy Living: *Asthma*

Jack Canfield

Mark Victor Hansen

Norman H. Edelman, M.D.

Health Communications, Inc.
Deerfield Beach, Florida

www.bcibooks.com
www.chickensoup.com

Library of Congress Cataloging-in-Publication Data
available from the Library of Congress

Publisher: Health Communications, Inc.
          3201 S.W. 15th Street
          Deerfield Beach, FL 33442–8190

Cover design by Larissa Hise Henoch
Inside book design by Lawna Patterson Oldfield
Inside book formatting by Dawn Von Strolley Grove

"This is something you live with your whole life.
Asthma's part of who I am,
and I can't control it if I don't know about it."

—CATHI B.

Contents

Fear less, hope more,

eat less, chew more,

whine less, breathe more,

talk less, say more,

love more,

and all good things

will be yours.

—Swedish Proverb

Introduction:
Breathe Easier with Asthma

Today, it seems as though asthma is everywhere. In fact, an estimated 20 million people—6.1 million of them children under 18—currently have asthma. If you are reading this book, then you know someone who suffers from this chronic disease. It could be you, a family member, a young child, a coworker, or a neighbor.

Asthma isn't always obvious; you can't tell an asthma sufferer from looking at them—unless they are having trouble breathing. Though you can't always see asthma, you can see and count its devastating effects. Asthma is the leading serious chronic illness among children. It is the number one cause of school absences attributed to chronic illnesses and accounts for a total of 14 million lost school days each year.

In every community, children and adults suffer from asthma, but in our inner cities, asthma is especially prevalent. In addition, although more prescriptions for asthma medications are being written, many people are not using their medications as prescribed. The result: an increase in asthma attacks that land people in the emergency room.

But the good news is that asthma in most cases *can* be controlled. Every person with asthma can and should expect to lead a normal life. Far too many people with asthma accept limitations on their life. Children accept the fact that they can't participate in gym class. Teenagers accept the fact that they can't do sports. Adults accept the fact that they have to get up twice a night almost every night, gasping for breath.

I want to reach people to make them understand that they should feel better and they can feel better. It's not okay to accept limitations on your life because of asthma. If asthma is holding you back, tell your doctor. Maybe your doctor can change your medication. Maybe you need to use an asthma inhaler before you exercise. Maybe you can make changes at home to get rid of asthma triggers.

One day, perhaps soon, we will be able not only to control asthma but to cure it. Today, there is great reason to hope for a cure for asthma. We have learned so much about asthma in recent years, particularly about the inflammation in the airways that leads to asthma. We have great reason to hope that we can eventually find the key to shutting off this inflammatory process and curing this disease.

But in the meantime, there are many things you

and your doctor can do to control your asthma so you can lead a healthy, normal life. On the following pages you'll learn many ways to control your asthma, like getting rid of asthma triggers in your home, having a plan that will tell you what to do in case you feel an asthma attack coming on, dealing with your child's asthma at home and at school, exercising with asthma, traveling with asthma, plus sections on asthma during the teen years, pregnancy and senior years.

I hope that you will come away from reading this book with tips that will help you or your loved one with asthma to breathe easier. The most important message I can give you about asthma is: you can control it—don't let it control you!

—Norman H. Edelman, M.D.
Chief Medical Officer
American Lung Association

Don't Let Asthma Control You!

Asthma. It means many things to many people. For some, asthma means wheezing during spring allergy season. For others, it means a daily struggle to breathe normally. Asthma affects people differently—some people have mild asthma, some severe.

But it's important for everyone with asthma and their families to know that you can control asthma—don't let it control you! If you're not breathing normally, don't accept it—it's not okay. This book will walk you through the steps you can take to begin to breathe normally again, in many situations, throughout your life.

Yes, most cases of asthma can be controlled. But unfortunately, many people with asthma continue to struggle with their breathing. Perhaps their asthma is being ignored in the hopes that it will simply go away. Or they aren't taking the right kind of medication. Or they aren't taking their medication as often as they should. Maybe they've been told—wrongly—that most people grow out of their asthma.

There are many reasons why people with asthma aren't breathing normally and aren't living life to the fullest. You don't have to be one of those people. You can—and should—live a normal, healthy life despite your asthma.

In fact, several Olympic medalists have had

asthma, including track and field star Jackie Joyner-Kersee and swimmer Tom Dolan. They are proof that asthma doesn't have to slow you down.

Famous People with Asthma

- Loni Anderson, actress
- Jason Alexander, actor, on "Seinfeld"
- Ludwig von Beethoven, composer
- Leonard Bernstein, conductor, composer
- Calvin Coolidge, thirtieth president of the United States
- Tom Dolan, Olympic medalist in swimming
- Morgan Fairchild, actress
- Bob Hope, comedian
- Jim "Catfish" Hunter, baseball player (Hall of Fame)
- John F. Kennedy, thirty-fifth president of the United States
- Jackie Joyner-Kersee, Olympic medalist in track and field
- Liza Minnelli, actress, singer
- Walter Mondale, forty-second vice president of the United States
- Dennis Rodman, basketball player
- Theodore Roosevelt, twenty-sixth president of the United States

- Elizabeth Taylor, actress
- Martin Van Buren, eighth president of the United States
- Dominique Wilkins, basketball player
- Woodrow Wilson, twenty-eighth president of the United States

The Littlest Gift

There was one surprising advantage to my first asthma attack, but it was entirely due to timing: I was five years old, it was Christmas Eve, and I wanted to see Santa Claus when he came to my house with the presents.

Every previous Christmas Eve, the excitement of the holidays had meant I hadn't a prayer of being able to stay awake and alert enough to see the big jolly man in red. This year, I would have given anything for the relief that sleep would have brought from the exhaustion of not being able to get enough air into my lungs. Still, I held out the faint hope that my wheezing wouldn't be too loud to eclipse the sound of sleigh bells and the hooves of eight reindeer on my roof.

My first asthma attack was precipitated by sitting too close to our church's nativity scene at Christmas Eve mass. To lend a little more authenticity to the scene that year, the church had hauled in bales of real hay and set up some plastic donkeys and horses. My parents thought it would be a harmless treat for me to sit close to the nativity scene so I could see better. I had always loved animals, but I had recently developed quite severe allergies to most of them, including cats and dogs. My parents hadn't counted on the hay itself triggering an allergy—they had logically assumed that if the animals were plastic, I was safe. They were wrong.

Halfway through Christmas Eve dinner, my nose started running, my eyes became red, itchy and watery, and I started coughing. Several hours later, I was in the full-blown horror of an asthma attack, and it was the most frightening thing that had ever happened to me. Every breath was a struggle, and it seemed that the harder I worked to get air in, the harder it became to breathe, and the more tired I became. It was like there was a heavy iron weight on my chest, squeezing all the air out of my lungs and taking away all my strength.

Shortly after midnight on Christmas morning, after a steam bath, hot tea, and allergy medicine had eased my symptoms but failed to cure them, it was clear that neither my mother nor I would be getting any sleep. She decided it was time to go to the hospital. I came out of the bathroom to see her arranging the presents under the tree. The room was dark but comforting, illuminated only by the gentle, cheerful colors of the Christmas tree lights. My eyes moved quickly to the plate of cookies, glass of milk, and carrots for the reindeer. Gone, all of them! I couldn't understand how I'd missed him. I'd been listening so hard. Then, as I watched my mother's quick movements with the logic and clarity of youth that inevitably leads to the first bloom of skepticism, it dawned on me. Maybe Santa Claus hadn't been here at all. I knew he was fast and clever, but how could he have waited until the exact moment when I went to the bathroom to deliver all those presents?

It was time to get this sorted out. "Hey, Mom," I croaked between wheezes, "What are you doing with those presents? Isn't that Santa's job?" I asked accusingly. "Well," she said calmly. "He's so busy that he just needed my help arranging them so they look pretty." I hesitated. This made sense, and she sounded sure of herself. Still, something didn't seem quite right.

"You can pick one present to open now and take with you to the hospital," she said gently but firmly. Still disgruntled at having missed the magical Santa Claus and growing crabbier by the minute, I picked the smallest package from the pile and was surprised when it made a little musical sound. I tore off the wrapping to reveal a miniature keyboard, not much wider or longer than the palm of my hand. I was instantly enchanted, and I did take it to the hospital with me, trying to concentrate on making familiar songs with its lovely delicate tones rather than my wheezing and exhaustion.

The little keyboard has long since lost its sound, but my asthma is much better. To this day, listening to any kind of music calms me in the midst of an attack. And my mother's real gift from that Christmas endures—she still does her best to shield me from disappointments, large and small, which I'm sure will never change.

♥ *Anne Stopper*

What Is Asthma?

Asthma is a disease that affects the airways in and out of the lungs. In a person with asthma, the airways are swollen or inflamed. They are very sensitive, and when you breathe in something irritating, or that you're allergic to, the airways narrow and become more inflamed.

The muscles around the outside of the airways also tighten up, making the airways even smaller. Cells in the airways make more mucus than usual, which also leads to narrower airways. The result of all these changes: less air gets to your lungs, which leads to wheezing, coughing, a feeling of chest tightness, and breathing difficulty. This is called an asthma attack, or episode.

Some asthma attacks are worse than others. In a severe asthma attack, the airways may become so narrow that the body is starved of oxygen, and the result can be deadly.

That is why it's so important to take asthma seriously. If you have asthma, visit your doctor regularly, avoid things that trigger your breathing problems, and take your medicines just the way your doctor tells you to. You'll be able to live life to the fullest and feel your best.

DIAGNOSING ASTHMA

A doctor diagnoses asthma based on a number of things, including your symptoms, family history of asthma and your breathing. As part of the exam, your doctor will use a device called a spirometer to check your airways. The spirometer measures how much air passes through the airways and how fast you can blow air out of your lungs after taking a deep breath. If you have asthma, the results will be lower than normal.

Depending on the results of your physical exam, medical history, and breathing tests, your doctor will figure out how severe your asthma is. The type of asthma you have determines how it should be treated. It's important to remember that a person with any type of asthma—even the mildest form—can still have asthma attacks. The four main categories of asthma are:

- **Mild intermittent (comes and goes)**—Your asthma is not well controlled, you have asthma symptoms twice a week or less and you are bothered by symptoms at night twice a month or less.
- **Mild persistent**—Your asthma is not well controlled and you have asthma symptoms more than twice a week, but no more than once in a single day. You are bothered by symptoms at

night more than twice a month. You may have
asthma attacks that affect your activity.

- **Moderate persistent**—Your asthma is not well
controlled, you have asthma symptoms every
day and you are bothered by nighttime symptoms more than once a week. Asthma attacks
may affect your activity.
- **Severe persistent**—Your asthma is not well
controlled, you have symptoms throughout the
day on most days and you are bothered by
nighttime symptoms often. In severe asthma,
your physical activity is likely to be limited.

When You First Hear the Word "Asthma"

Hearing from your doctor that you or a family
member has asthma may bring on some strong
emotions. You may not want to believe it's true.
You might be scared, anxious or depressed. Those
feelings are all normal.

Once you accept that you or your loved one
has asthma, you can start taking steps to control
your breathing. Working with your doctor, you
will learn how to identify and control asthma
triggers and take asthma medicine to prevent
asthma attacks. You'll have an asthma action plan
to tell you exactly what to do if you feel your
breathing start to change.

The more you learn about your asthma, the more confidence you'll have in your ability to manage any breathing problems that may arise. You'll avoid unnecessary hospital visits, and be able to let go of those feelings of distress.

Allergies and Asthma

While you or your child may have asthma but not allergies, or allergies but not asthma, many people have both conditions together. Eczema (allergic skin inflammation) and hay fever are the two most common allergies that people with asthma have. If you suffer from hay fever and you have asthma, you know only too well the feeling of a runny nose and watery eyes combined with the wheezing and coughing that signal an asthma attack.

Mold, dust mites, animal dander and cockroaches can also cause allergic symptoms in the nose and eyes while causing asthma symptoms in the airways.

Think about . . .
my asthma attitude

These are the things asthma keeps me from doing:

_____

_____

_____

I wish I didn't have asthma because:

_____

_____

_____

If I was never bothered by asthma, I would:

_____

_____

_____

Something I've learned from having asthma is:

_____

_____

_____

The Angry Elephant

An angry elephant is sitting on my chest. When I struggle to breathe, the elephant only presses harder, closing off my airways, making each breath more difficult than the last.

The elephant's name is asthma.

Usually, the elephant leaves me alone. I run around waiting on tables at my restaurant job without getting winded. I play tennis, hike and practice yoga. I laugh and quarrel with my husband and gossip with my girlfriends. Most of the time, I'm just another middle-age woman who worries about money, loves her family, and wonders what it might be like to kiss Brad Pitt.

Without warning, I catch a nasty cold that turns into a stubborn cough followed by a tightness in my chest, and an inability to talk without wheezing. My lungs feel as if they are full of glue.

Removing that elephant off my chest is all that matters. I don't worry about wrinkles or credit card bills or squabbles at my job. Each labored breath is more precious than the last. When my asthma gets

out of control, I'm reminded that the nasty elephant is still on my chest. Since I was diagnosed
with asthma 20 years ago, I've been hospitalized
twice, not counting several emergency room visits
and countless sleepless nights gasping for air.

And yet I sometimes still have trouble admitting
I have asthma.

Growing up, everyone called me the healthy
child, the one who danced through life never out of
breath. It was different for my mother and little
brother. My mother wore a medical alert bracelet
identifying her as an asthma patient. One bee sting
could trigger an allergic reaction and an asthma
attack. My little brother had to drink syruplike, bit-
ter medicine and sleep in a cloud of vaporized
steam to keep his lungs open.

I was the strong, free girl while my mother and
brother were imprisoned with sensitive, sick lungs.
They had allergies that might trigger asthma while
I could rub my face in a cat's fur without my eyes
watering. I played all day in a field of flowers and
tall grasses without worrying about pollen. Dust
only made me sneeze, not wheeze. When I caught a
cold, I didn't have to be rushed to the doctor like my
brother.

While dealing with their asthma, neither my
mother nor my little brother ever complained, or
acted sorry for themselves or were afraid it might

kill them. They both just accepted that it was part of who they were, like having blue eyes or an outward belly button. I often reflect on my childhood and admire how bravely my mother and brother lived with asthma during a time when there weren't many advanced medications.

I was the one who whined about asthma. Why couldn't we have a cat? Or goose-down pillows? Why did my mother have to spend my seventh birthday party in a hospital bed? Why did we have to cut short our vacation to Canada just because my brother was wheezing?

During my early twenties, I moved away from home and put my family's asthma behind me. I smoked cigarettes, worked in smoky nightclubs, slept on feather pillows in dusty rooms and took my lungs for granted as I always had.

Then, when I was 29, my genetic time clock kicked in. I always was the late bloomer. Part of me was glad I escaped asthma as a child, and the other half of me refused to truly accept the doctor's diagnosis.

I didn't like to tell friends for fear they might view me as "weak." It embarrassed me to use my inhaler in public. I took my doctor's advice and medication haphazardly. I told people I didn't mind if they smoked in my house. I'd wait until that elephant was stomping on me before I'd seek help and then become impatient when the doctor couldn't "fix me" immediately.

I wanted to pretend I was still that little girl with the perfect lungs who only watched other people have asthma. All I could see was what was taken from me and not what was given, the opportunity to take better care of my body.

With age comes many things, but especially the understanding that immortality is reserved for people in white robes with wings. Besides, the mirror won't let me pretend I'm a little girl anymore. Breathing matters more than other people's opinions.

As I inch closer to 50, my angry elephant and I have finally come to an agreement. I take my medications, get plenty of rest, don't smoke, avoid air pollutants and get exercise. I go to the doctor without shame.

Asthma has taught me I must accept my weakness to truly be strong.

♥ *Susanne Brent*

Asthma Triggers

A person with asthma has his or her own set of asthma "triggers." These are things that can set off a reaction in your lungs that can lead to an asthma attack. Triggers can be found indoors or outdoors. Check off the triggers that make your asthma worse:

___ Cold air
___ Tobacco smoke
___ Exercise
___ Wood smoke
___ Perfume
___ Paint
___ Hair spray
___ Other strong odors or fumes
___ Dust mites
___ Pollen
___ Molds
___ Pollution
___ Animal dander (tiny scales or particles that fall off hair, feathers or skin of pets)
___ Common cold, flu or other respiratory diseases
___ Other (fill in here)_____

It's not always easy to figure out what your

triggers are. If you do know what they are, cutting down your exposure to them may help you avoid asthma attacks.

If you don't know your triggers, try picking one or two on the list above and limiting your exposure to them. See if your asthma gets better. This may indicate these are triggers for your asthma.

IN YOUR HOME

Some people with asthma find their symptoms get worse at night. If you're one of these people, try sleeping with air conditioning. Because you keep the windows and doors closed, you're keeping pollen and mold spores outside. Air conditioning also lowers the humidity indoors, which helps control mold and dust mites.

The following are tips for controlling common triggers:

Tobacco smoke. Don't allow smoking in your home. Ask family members and guests to smoke outside. Even better, suggest they quit smoking!

Cockroaches. Small pieces of the insects and their droppings end up in house dust, and from there, into the air you breathe. To get rid of roaches:

- Store food in sealable containers and keep crumbs, dirty dishes and other food cleaned up.
- Fix leaks and wipe up standing water.

• If you choose to use a pesticide, consider baits—they're less likely than sprays or foggers to harm your lungs.

Indoor mold. Bathrooms, kitchens and basements are prime spots for mold when humidity is high.

• Make sure air circulation is good in these areas, and the areas are cleaned often.
• Consider a dehumidifier for the basement—empty the water and clean the container often to prevent mildew.
• Wash foam pillows every week to get rid of mold that may form from perspiration. Dry them thoroughly and change them once a year.
• Check houseplants for mold. You may need to keep plants outdoors.

Strong odors or fumes. Avoid or use very sparingly:

• Perfume
• Room deodorizers
• Talcum powder
• Paint
• Cleaning chemicals

Dust mites. These tiny, microscopic spiders are found in house dust. One pinch of dust may have several thousand mites.

- Put mattresses in dust-proof, allergen-impermeable covers, and tape over the zipper.
- Put pillows in allergen-impermeable covers, and tape over the zipper. Or wash the pillow every week.
- Wash all bedding every week in water that is at least 130° F. Removing the bedspread at night may help.
- Don't sleep or lie down on upholstered furniture.
- Get rid of carpeting in the bedroom.
- Clean up dust as often as you can, using a damp mop or damp cloth. Don't use aerosols or spray cleaners in the bedroom. And don't clean when someone with asthma is in the room.
- To avoid dust on window coverings, use window shades or curtains made of plastic or other washable material for easy cleaning.
- Remove stuffed furniture and stuffed animals (unless the animals can be washed), and anything under the bed.
- Closets are a big source of dust mites. Try putting clothes in a plastic garment bag (not the plastic bag that covers dry cleaning).
- Get a dehumidifier because dust mites like moisture and high humidity.
- Try a vacuum with a high efficiency filter or a central vacuum that blows dust and other allergens outside the home.

Pets and Asthma

It can be devastating to a family to find out that a family member's asthma is triggered by a beloved pet. Dogs and cats can trigger asthma problems, but so can other animals, like birds, guinea pigs or hamsters. Doctors recommend that the pet in question be removed from the home when it triggers asthma, but that's not an easy decision to make. What should you do?

If you do decide to remove the pet, it's important to know that pet allergen remains in house dust and may continue to trigger asthma symptoms even after the pet is gone. Clean the house—especially carpets and upholstered furniture—thoroughly. If you are looking to get a new pet, try tropical fish.

It's also important to explain to children that the pet is being removed for important health reasons. Children in the household who don't have asthma may feel resentful about losing their pet and blame the person with asthma. Explaining that the pet can cause serious breathing problems for a person with asthma may help the child to understand why the family has made this difficult decision.

If you decide to keep the pet, there are measures you can take to help cut down on the amount of allergen that is spread through the house. But no matter what you do, animal allergen will still be in the air and carried on the clothing of people in your home, so you'll still be exposing the person with asthma to allergens.

Ways to cut down on animal allergens in the home include:

- Keeping pets out of the bedroom of the person with asthma and keeping the door closed.
- Keeping pets away from carpets, fabric-covered furniture and stuffed toys.
- Vacuuming carpets, rugs and furniture two or more times every week.

Think about . . .
cutting down on asthma triggers

A big change I can make is to:

_____

_____

_____

An easy change I can make is to:

_____

_____

_____

When I'm cleaning I will:

_____

_____

_____

I'll get rid of:

_____

_____

_____

I'll ask family members to:

_____

_____

_____

The Air Quality Index

Those hazy days of summer can be hard on the lungs of people with asthma. That's because ozone, the primary ingredient of smog air pollution, is very harmful to breathe. Luckily, you can find out at the beginning of each day how bad the air is, and plan accordingly, with the help of a very handy tool—the Air Quality Index, or AQI. This is the system that state and local air pollution control programs use to notify the public about levels of air pollution.

In most cities and suburbs, air pollution levels are measured daily and ranked on a scale of 0 for the cleanest air all the way up to 500 for air pollution levels that pose immediate danger to the public. The AQI further breaks air pollution levels into five categories, each of which has a name, color and advisory statement.

How Do You Find Air Quality Information?

• Air quality forecasts may be included as part of your local weather forecast on TV and radio, or printed in the newspaper. AQI levels are also available online, through local agencies and the U.S. Environmental Protection Agency (EPA) (*www.epa.gov/airnow*).

- State and local air pollution control agencies are responsible for collecting air quality data and reporting the AQI. You can call them for current information if it is not available through the media. A directory of state and local agencies is available from STAPPA/ALAPCO, their national membership association, at *www.cleanairworld.org.*

- The EPA issues year-round AQI forecasts for 46 states plus the District of Columbia. Forecasts include animated pictures of ozone and particle pollution levels superimposed over a map of the United States. The map illustrates how pollution levels change and move throughout the day. It is "real time" information, so you can see current outdoor air quality. The map is available at *www.epa.gov/airnow.*

Breathing to Death

It was stupid. But at the time the whole thing made perfect sense to me. I had convinced myself that I was going to cure myself of asthma.

I used to ask my doctor for a cure. He always laughed at me. I am the kind of person who makes people laugh, so when I asked for a cure, he thought I was joking.

I wasn't joking. When I told the doctor that someday I was going to just throw all the medicine out and let this asthma cure itself, I wasn't joking either. I wanted to get rid of asthma like an old coat. I was tired of sewing on patches. The patches looked ugly and the coat wasn't keeping me warm anymore.

Having had asthma from childhood and having lived through this miracle cure and that miracle cure, I guess I had just overdosed on being a pill-inhaler-steroid-dependent. I was tired of hearing about all the people with "seasonal asthma" who were getting relief from some new pill that was making springtime poetic. I was sick of hearing about people with "exercised-induced asthma" getting relief from some new inhaler used before swimming 900 miles at top speed.

I was having problems sleeping through the night and walking through the supermarket; the new drugs weren't doing a thing for me.

I was living in the nineties. People were jogging to the mall and aerobic kickboxing their way into the twenty-first century. I couldn't get from one end of my house to the other without using an inhaler. And the inhaler didn't always work, so the doctor was pumping me up with prednisone, a drug that was causing me to gain weight. And I was living on the stuff.

Because of my asthma, we moved from New York to Arizona, where, at the time, they said the air was cleaner and drier. In Arizona I might have a better chance at good health. We got off the plane along with a half million other people, and these other people all had cars that helped pollute the desert air and they lived in houses with swimming pools which each added to the overall humidity level. And they told two friends. And so on. And so on. Arizona was not the answer.

I was already in a mild depression from living a life where I had to think about what I could and couldn't do. People with the best intentions were always asking me why I wasn't taking the pill that so-and-so was taking and getting relief from. If so-and-so could win a gold medal in the Olympics, I certainly had no excuses for restricting my activities.

So I threw out my medicine. I threw out the inhalers and the pills. I threw out the breathing machine and the gadget that helped me measure my breathing effectiveness. I threw out the doctor's phone number. I threw it all out.

The fatal error is that I almost killed myself in the process of trying to cure myself. My body shut down totally. I stopped breathing. I was curled up on the floor with my husband screaming into the phone for 911 to send help, with my sons staring down at me, crying, "Don't let Mommy die!"

Then the ambulance came and they got me to the hospital. I was hooked up to machines. The doctors pumped me up with this and that. I don't remember most of it. And three days later in intensive care, my doctor was scratching his head saying, "You were serious?"

The truth was that I was seriously depressed, and no one recognized it.

I'd been putting up that false medicated front for so long that recognizing it might have been impossible. I'd spent a lifetime of sitting away from everyone who was sitting in the grass because the grass made me wheeze. I spent a life of not having friends with pets because I couldn't visit them. I spent a life of avoiding foods and activities and places. We saved for years and went to Hawaii. Everyone went scuba diving. I held the towels. I fretted through two pregnancies of taking life-sustaining medicines in spite of the potential damage to the fetuses. Friends were afraid to take an aspirin for a headache when they were pregnant; I lived on mass quantities of medicines through both pregnancies, worrying constantly of potential side effects the medicines were going to have. Two healthy children later, my asthma kept getting worse.

There was a time when I could predict an attack. Now the attacks were coming without signs. And I was taking a ton of drugs that were helping me mildly, but not enough to allow me a normal existence.

My doctor became wiser after seeing me in intensive care. If he had passed me off to a therapist, I don't think I would have gained control of my asthma and ultimately, regained control of my life. I don't think until this time he quite understood the level of depression that I was suffering because of my asthma. I think I scared him. And more important, I scared myself.

A few weeks after the night in the emergency room, the doctor called me. He told me a new medicine was being released. This time it was my turn to be lucky. It worked.

I'm not a doctor, but I am an expert on my own asthma. And as an expert, it scares me that death can be as simple as a breath away, and it empowers me knowing that I've gained control of my life and my greatest fear.

♥ *Felice Prager*

Take Charge of Your Health Care

While it is up to you to determine the ways to deal with and treat your asthma, having a strong relationship with your doctor will help you make the best choice. Your doctor can help you figure out how to deal with your symptoms and how to work with you to help you breathe easier.

Make a list of your questions before you visit the doctor and feel free to refer to the list during your visit. If your doctor says anything you don't understand, ask to have it repeated. If doctor visits tend to overwhelm you, bring along a friend or relative who can take notes, offer support and help ask questions.

Tell your doctor about:

Any herbs or dietary supplements you're taking. Just because you can buy them without a prescription doesn't mean they're harmless.

Your symptoms. Describe your symptoms: when they started, how they make you feel, what triggers them and what you've done to relieve them.

Your daily habits. Don't be embarrassed—be honest about your diet, physical activity, smoking and alcohol or drug use. Your doctor can't give you the best care if you withhold information.

Ask about:

• **Test results**—how will you find out about

them and how long it will take to get them.
- **Side effects** of any medication you've been pre-scribed. Are there alternatives? How much will it cost, how long will it last and will insurance cover it?
- **How to take the medicine:** what to do if you miss a dose; if there are any foods, drugs or activities you should avoid when taking the medicine; and if there is a generic brand available at a lower price—you can ask your pharmacist these questions, too.

GETTING A SECOND OPINION

There are times when you may not feel comfortable with a particular doctor. Don't dismiss those feelings. If you don't feel at ease talking with that person, you may want to consider switching doctors.

Or you may not agree with your doctor's recommendations. In that case, you should think about getting a second opinion. Another doctor might have a different perspective or new options for treatment and give you new information.

Here are some tips on how to get a second opinion:

- Ask your doctor to recommend someone else—either another primary care doctor or a specialist—for another opinion. Don't worry about hurting your doctor's feelings. If you prefer, you can call a university hospital or medical society in your area for names of doctors.

- Check with your health insurance provider to see if they cover the cost of a second opinion, and make sure the person you're going to is covered under the plan. Find out if you need a referral from your primary care doctor.

- Have your primary care doctor send medical records to the doctor you're seeing for a second opinion so you don't have to repeat any medical tests. Your primary care doctor's office may charge a fee for this service.

- As with your primary care doctor, come prepared to meet the new doctor with a list of questions and concerns.

- Ask this doctor to send a written report to your primary care doctor, and get a copy for your own records.

*"I tell patients, 'If you brought your car
in to the mechanic and you picked it up
and it clunked out of the parking lot,
you'd go back in and demand that it be fixed.
You need to do that with your asthma.'"*

—LEROY GRAHAM, M.D., PEDIATRIC PULMONOLOGIST

Beating Asthma

It was my first year at summer camp, and I was excited and scared, but more important, I was alone. I had taken a plane to Wisconsin, hundreds of miles away from my home, to spend three long weeks away from my parents.

A few days later, I was in love with camp. I enjoyed all the different activities, from swimming in the lake to eating with my cabin mates in the big mess hall.

One day, I was very late to dinner and I was scared that I would get in trouble with my counselors. I loved all of them and I desperately wanted to be a great camper. I dashed out of my cabin, slammed the screen door and started running across camp. As I ran I felt my chest start to coil tighter and tighter, but

I was in too much of a hurry to stop and worry about it. As I stopped in front of the mess hall, I noticed there was a squeaky sound coming from my chest and that it was very hard to breathe. As I went into the mess hall and sat down, I just kept trying to ignore it, but my breathing was getting worse.

Finally, I gathered my courage and went up to my youngest counselor, Laura. I sat down on the bench next to her and said, "Laura, I can't breathe." She looked really surprised and I could tell she couldn't quite believe me. She told me to put my head on her lap and concentrate on breathing. But my breathing was getting worse and I was starting to panic.

At last, Laura helped me up and we started walking across camp to the infirmary. As we walked, I vaguely remember Laura talking to me and telling me to keep breathing, but I was so terrified, the walk was a blur. When we got to the infirmary, the doctor put a mask over my face and told me to breathe deeply. Finally I could breathe! When the treatment was over, the doctor sat down next to me and said, "Emily, I think you have asthma, I am going to order you an inhaler and it will be here tomorrow." I was sure he was kidding. Me, have asthma? No way! But he said it was true.

The next day, as I came to realize my fate, I was terrified. Here I was, hundreds of miles from home, and the scariest thing that had ever happened to me was happening without my parents. My counselors tried to be there for me, but I was miserable, and sick too. That summer I spent more time in the infirmary than out.

At last I came home, and my asthma was confirmed through breathing tests. My asthma is now well controlled with the help of steroids, and I have the support I need from my parents and friends. I am so proud of myself, because I know I am beating asthma.

♥ *Emily Bamberger*

Treat Your Asthma

The type of asthma medicines you take depend on how severe your asthma is and other factors. These medicines keep the airways open. Asthma medicines are sold under many brand names and come in many forms, including sprays, pills, powders, liquids and shots. No one drug is best for every kind of asthma or every person. You and your doctor need to work together to find the best medicines and the right amounts for you.

When your asthma is properly treated, it should be controlled, and you should not have asthma symptoms. If you are taking asthma medicine and you still have trouble breathing, don't just assume this is "normal" for you. It's not! Tell your doctor what your symptoms are and when you have them. Then you can work with your doctor to find the right medicine or combination of medicines to keep your asthma under control.

MEDICATIONS

There are two main types of medications for asthma:

Quick relief medicines are taken when your asthma symptoms are getting worse and you may be on your way to having an asthma attack. These medicines start working within minutes to prevent an asthma attack.

You use quick relief medicines only when needed. A common type of quick relief medicine is a **short-acting, inhaled bronchodilator**. Bronchodilators relax tightened muscles around the airways. They help open up airways quickly and make breathing easier. Although these medicines act quickly, they only last for a short time. You should take quick relief medicines when you *first* begin to feel asthma symptoms like coughing, wheezing, chest tightness or shortness of breath. You should always have a quick-relief inhaler in case of an attack. Your doctor may also suggest that you use your quick-relief inhaler before you exercise.

Long-term control medicines are taken every day, usually for a long period of time, to control ongoing symptoms and to prevent asthma attacks. It usually takes a few weeks before you feel the full effects of these medicines. If you have persistent asthma, you'll need long-term control medicines.

- **Inhaled corticosteroids** are the most effective long-term control medications for asthma. This medicine reduces the swelling of airways that makes asthma attacks more likely. Inhaled steroids are recommended for mild, moderate and severe persistent asthma. Your doctor will show you how to correctly use the inhaler. In some cases, steroids are given in tablet or liquid form for a short time to bring asthma under control, or for a longer time to control severe asthma.

- **Long-acting beta-agonists** help control moderate and severe asthma and prevent nighttime symptoms. Long-acting beta-agonists are taken together with inhaled corticosteroids.
- **Leukotriene modifiers** are used either alone to treat mild persistent asthma or together with inhaled corticosteroids to treat moderate persistent asthma or severe persistent asthma.
- **Cromolyn** and **nedocromil** are used to treat mild persistent asthma.
- **Theophylline** is used either alone to treat mild persistent asthma or together with inhaled corticosteroids to treat moderate persistent asthma. People who take theophylline should have their blood levels checked to be sure they are taking a safe dose.

Many people with asthma need both a short-acting bronchodilator to use when their symptoms get worse and long-term, daily asthma control medication to treat the underlying inflammation of the airways that causes asthma.

Think about . . .
my asthma medicines

Here are the asthma medicines I take:

Name	Dose	How often I take it	Why I take it

Side Effects

If you have any of the following side effects, tell your doctor—he or she may change the dose or try a different medicine:

- Sore throat
- Nervousness
- Nausea
- Rapid heartbeat
- Loss of appetite
- Staying awake

Think about . . .
my health checklist

Work with Your Doctor

Go through this checklist before you visit the doctor, and be sure to share your answers with the doctor.

Since my last visit:

My asthma is worse.	___YES ___NO
I've had changes in my home, work or school environment (such as a new pet or someone smoking).	___YES ___NO
At least one time, my symptoms were a lot worse than usual.	___YES ___NO
My asthma has caused me to miss work or school or reduce or change my activities.	___YES ___NO
I've missed any regular doses of my medicines.	___YES ___NO
My medications have caused me problems (shakiness, nervousness, bad taste, sore throat, cough, upset stomach).	___YES ___NO

I've had an emergency room visit
or hospital stay for asthma.   ___YES ___NO

The cost of my asthma treatment
has kept me from getting the
medicine or care I need for my
asthma.   ___YES ___NO

I have increased how often I
take quick-relief asthma
medicine.   ___YES ___NO

I have woken up at night more
often because of my asthma.   ___YES ___NO

Get a Flu Shot

If you have asthma, you should get a flu shot.
The flu, or influenza, can cause an asthma attack
and poses a major health risk to people with
asthma. For some people, a flu-induced asthma
attack is serious enough to require a trip to the
emergency room. A study conducted by the
American Lung Association found the flu shot
will not cause an asthma attack in children and
adults with asthma.

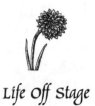

Life Off Stage

The diagnosis was frightening. How could I be so healthy one day and, weeks later, be receiving the news I had asthma? The American Lung Association once said, and to me it is all too true, "If you can't breathe, nothing else matters." I had never felt grateful for my breathing until now.

I wasn't aggressive about seeking medical help. Being a successful, healthy dance studio owner, I believed that I could control most things. I would allow only two or three days away from work, no matter what the illness. I felt irreplaceable. Being dependent, needy and vulnerable for weeks, then months, was a truth I couldn't grasp.

Life now revolved around my nebulizer, a compressor for dispensing inhaled steroids, my many bottles of medicine and wishing life would be as it once was.

Who was I if I couldn't perform my roles as business person, wife, mother, grandmother? What was my purpose? Exhausted continually, I had been forced off the stage of my life.

A trip to a large medical center presented me with my first hope: a doctor who spoke encouraging words about treatments for asthma. She pressed her stethoscope to my chest as I struggled to inhale, lungs burning. The exhale, even without a stethoscope, produced a squeaking, whistling sound, very familiar to me by then. She wrote me prescriptions and we scheduled a follow-up visit.

Time and medication began to restore my breathing and my energy. I still have asthma. But my asthma has made me appreciate more fully life's gifts: I witnessed the birth of my granddaughter on a chilly summer morning in Alaska, I celebrated my birthday with my husband from a hot air balloon, I made sandcastles with my grandchildren, I cheered for my sister as she became a pilot, I loved more deeply than I thought possible.

This life off stage has brought gratitude, an awareness of my blessings and richness far beyond anything material. Today, I live with intention, looking forward, making decisions based on a "no regrets" criteria. I no longer ask myself who I am off stage. The answer clearly lies in who and what I love.

♥ *Vicki Armitage*

Get an Asthma Action Plan!

When you or a family member has asthma, you have a lot to keep track of. That's why every person with asthma needs an asthma action plan. The plan is written by your doctor to help you manage your asthma. It tells you what to do based on changes in your symptoms and your peak flow numbers (see peak flow meter section below).

An asthma action plan is especially important in an emergency. Keep copies of it handy, and make sure it's current. Review it with your doctor at least once a year.

USE A PEAK FLOW METER

To help you measure your lung function, your doctor may give you a handheld device called a peak flow meter to use at home. To use it, you take a deep breath and blow hard into a tube to find out how fast you can blow out. This gives you a peak flow number. You find out your "personal best" by writing down the peak flow number daily for a few weeks until your asthma is under control. The highest number you get during that time is your personal best peak flow. You can compare future peak flow measurements to your personal best peak flow, and that will show if your asthma is under control.

Your doctor will tell you how and when to use

your peak flow meter and how to use your medicine based on the results. The peak flow meter can help warn of a possible asthma attack even before you notice any symptoms. If your peak flow meter shows that your breathing is getting worse, you should follow your action plan.

WHAT'S MY NORMAL PEAK FLOW RATE?

Peak flow rates are usually broken down into three zones: green, yellow and red.

Green Zone:

Eighty to 100 percent of your usual or "normal" peak flow rate means all clear. A reading in this zone means that your asthma is under reasonably good control—just keep following the asthma management program your doctor has recommended.

Yellow Zone:

Fifty to 80 percent of your usual or "normal" peak flow rate means caution. Your airways are narrowing and may require extra treatment. Your symptoms can get better or worse depending on what you do, or how and when you use your prescribed medication. You and your doctor should have a plan for yellow zone readings.

Red Zone:

Less than 50 percent of your usual or "normal" peak flow rate means a medical alert. You may be experiencing severe airway narrowing. Take your rescue medications right away. Contact your doctor now and follow the plan he or she has given you for red zone readings.

We suggest you have a written, easily located asthma action plan in your house. To download the American Lung Association Asthma Action Plan, visit *www.lungusa.org* and type "asthma action plan" in the search box.

ASTHMA ACTION PLAN

Work with your doctor to fill out this information.

General Information:

Name_____

Emergency Contact_____

Phone Numbers _____

Physician/Health Care Provider _____

Phone Numbers _____

Severity of Asthma

__Mild Intermittent

__Mild Persistent

__Moderate Persistent

__Severe Persistent

Triggers

__Colds

__Exercise

__Animals

__Smoke

__Dust

__Food

__Weather

__Air pollution

__Other_____

Exercise

1. Premedication (how much and when)

2. Exercise modifications _____

_____

GREEN ZONE: Doing Well

Peak Flow Meter Personal Best=_____

Symptoms

• Breathing is good

• No cough or wheeze

• Can work and play

• Sleeps all night

Control Medications

Medicine	How Much to Take	When to Take It
_____	_____	_____
_____	_____	_____
_____	_____	_____

Peak Flow Meter

More than 80 percent of personal best or _____

_____

YELLOW ZONE: Getting Worse

Contact physician if using quick relief medicines
more than two times per week.

Symptoms
- Some problems breathing
- Cough, wheeze or chest tight
- Problems working or playing
- Wake at night

Peak Flow Meter
Between 50 to 80 percent of personal best or
_____ to _____

Continue control medications and add:

Medicine	How Much to Take	When to Take It
_____	_____	_____
_____	_____	_____
_____	_____	_____

IF your symptoms (and peak flow, if used) return to Green Zone after one hour of the quick relief treatment, THEN

__ Take quick-relief medication every four hours for one to two days

__ Change your long-term control medicines by

_____

__ Contact your physician for follow-up care

**IF your symptoms (and peak flow, if used)
DO NOT return to the GREEN ZONE after
one hour of the quick relief treatment, THEN**

__ Take quick-relief treatment again

__ Change your long-term control medicines by

_____

__ Call your physician/health care provider
within__hours of modifying your medication
routine _____

_____

RED ZONE: Medical Alert

Ambulance/Emergency Phone Number:

Symptoms:

• Lots of problems breathing

• Cannot work or play

• Getting worse instead of better

• Medicine is not helping

Peak Flow Meter

Between 0 to 50 percent of personal best or ___

_____ to _____

Continue control medications and add:

Medicine	How Much to Take	When to Take It
_____	_____	_____
_____	_____	_____
_____	_____	_____

Go to the hospital or call for an ambulance if
__ Still in the red zone after fifteen minutes
__ If you have not been able to reach your
   physician/health care provider for help
__ Other _____

Call an ambulance immediately if the following
danger signs are present:

__ Trouble walking/talking due to shortness of
   breath
__ Lips or fingernails are blue

Disney Dreams

I was diagnosed with asthma at a very exciting time in my life. I had just been accepted as a performer at a major theme park in the United States. Now it seemed that my dream was unlikely to come true.

As an athletic college student, my sudden breathing problems came as a big surprise. The road to diagnosis was a bumpy one. At my lowest moment, I could not even walk across my college campus without getting out of breath. I couldn't understand how a seemingly healthy person could develop this kind of chronic disease overnight. How was I ever going to be able to perform in a theme park when I couldn't even walk across campus? It didn't seem possible. I didn't know anybody who had asthma, and I felt very alone. I was referred to a very good physician, who was able to help me start on the path of my new life.

I found out that not only did I have asthma, I also had allergies that triggered my asthma. By getting my allergies under control, I was able to get my asthma under control. I was able to start working out for the first time since I had started school, and it finally seemed like my dream of performing would once again be a reality.

As I geared up for the possibility of being a performer, I engaged in a lot of prayer and soul searching. I worried whether I would be able to handle the physical nature of my new job, especially in light of my new diagnosis. With the help of some good friends at my campus's Catholic Newman Center who supported me during this turbulent time in my life, my family and two very good doctors, my dream is now a reality. I perform in up to three parades a day in the extreme heat, and while having asthma means it is not always easy, it has made my victory that much sweeter.

My new goal for myself is to become more physically active and one day participate in the Danskin Women's Triathlon at Walt Disney World, a feat that seemed impossible even before my diagnosis. When I was first diagnosed with asthma, I would never have dreamed of setting my sights on such a goal. I know now, however, that with a little prayer and determination, I can do anything. Who knows? Perhaps one day I will see you at the finish line.

♥ *Jessica Berger*

When Your Asthma Isn't Under Control

If your asthma doesn't seem to be getting better even though you are taking steps to control it, don't be discouraged. Here are some possibilities to explore with your doctor:

- **Something in my home is triggering my asthma.** Reread the section on asthma triggers in this book, and think about whether any of the common asthma triggers—dust mites, pet dander, cockroaches, mold or tobacco smoke, for example—could be triggering your symptoms.
- **Something in my workplace is triggering my asthma.** Do some of your coworkers also have asthma symptoms at work? Does your breathing improve on weekends or vacations? If so, your doctor can help you figure out what the trigger might be, and if you can avoid it.
- **I'm not taking my medication correctly.** Go over the medication plan that your doctor has given you to make sure you're following it exactly.
- **I'm not using my inhaler the right way.** If you don't use your inhaler correctly, you're probably not getting enough medicine into your lungs. Ask your doctor if you need a spacer, a

device that helps more of the medicine get deeper into your lungs. Your doctor will show you how to use a spacer correctly.

- **I may need to change medicines.** If the medicines you're taking aren't controlling your asthma, you may need to change them. For instance, you may need to take one long-term controller medicine every day to fight inflammation in the lungs, and also take a quick-relief medicine to deal with asthma symptoms.

- **I don't know when my asthma is getting bad.** You may need to use a peak flow meter several times a day to monitor how well your lungs are working. Keeping track of your peak flow can tell you if you may need to take extra medicine or call your doctor. Your doctor will teach you how to use a peak flow meter and how to interpret the results.

- **I may have medical triggers such as GERD (heartburn with reflux) or chronic sinusitis.** Up to 70 percent of people with asthma have GERD compared with 20 percent to 30 percent of the general population. If you have severe, chronic asthma that does not respond well to treatment, you are even more susceptible to GERD. Sinusitis also is common in people with asthma.

- **Maybe I don't really have asthma.** If you've

followed all your doctor's instructions and still are having problems, perhaps you have another illness that acts like asthma. Your doctor may want to do other tests to make sure you really have asthma.

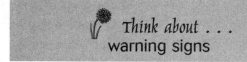

Think about . . .
warning signs

Do you have any of these signs? It might mean your asthma is not under control:

___ My asthma symptoms are occurring more often.

___ My asthma symptoms are worse than they used to be.

___ My asthma symptoms are bothering me a lot at night and making me lose sleep.

___ My asthma is causing me to miss work.

___ My child's asthma is causing him or her to miss school.

___ My peak flow number is low or varies a lot from morning to evening.

___ My asthma medications do not seem to be working very well anymore.

___ I have to use my short-acting, quick relief or rescue inhaler more often. (Using quick relief medicine every day, or using more than one inhaler a month is too much.)

___ I have had to go to the emergency room or doctor's because of an asthma attack.

___ I have ended up in the hospital because of my asthma.

Asthma Can't Smash Olympic Ambitions

I was diagnosed when I was 18, a freshman at UCLA, and we didn't know exactly what was going on. But I was doing a lot of wheezing and had shortness of breath and had been misdiagnosed with bronchitis. Finally, I went to an allergist, and they said I had asthma. And from there, we started working on trying to recognize my triggers, as well as the symptoms.

When I was having the shortness of breath, I thought mainly I was out of shape, and I was afraid UCLA was going to take my scholarship away. And then, once I was diagnosed, I was living in denial. I didn't want to believe that I had asthma, so I wasn't doing the things they were telling me to do to really get my asthma under control.

The key is controlling and managing your asthma, making sure you get your lung function test. It's very important for you to educate yourself on your medication, working with your doctor so you can control your asthma and stop living in denial. After you do that test, go over those results with your doctor. It could tell you where you are and then start following a program to start better controlling your asthma. Because asthma shouldn't control you. You should be controlling it. And that's the one thing I had to do, because at one particular time, asthma was controlling me.

♥ *Jackie Joyner-Kersee*, six-time Olympic medalist, from National Public Radio interview with Tavis Smiley

Asthma and Exercise

Some people with asthma begin wheezing and breathing harder after they exercise, or after they run up stairs or carry heavy things. This is called exercise-induced asthma.

Unfortunately, many people with exercise-induced asthma simply stop exercising because they want to avoid asthma attacks. But then they become out of shape, and even more likely to have breathing problems when they do anything strenuous.

Don't let asthma stop you from exercising! The benefits of exercise are too great to miss. Exercising reduces your risk of heart disease, helps you lose weight, makes you look and feel great, reduces stress . . . the list goes on and on.

The trick is to choose the kinds of exercise that are least likely to cause breathing problems, and to work with your doctor to see if you need to take medicine before exercising to avoid having an asthma attack.

Signs of exercise-induced asthma include breathing trouble (wheezing, chest tightness, coughing or chest pain) within 5 to 20 minutes after exercise. In some people, asthma symptoms start after they stop exercising. Cold air, air pollution, high pollen counts and colds all can worsen the effects of exercise-induced asthma.

If you think you may have exercise-induced asthma, ask your doctor. He or she can do a breathing test while you exercise to see if you indeed have this problem.

The best activities for people with exercise-induced asthma include

- Swimming
- Walking
- Leisure biking
- Hiking

When exercising outdoors in cold weather, wear a scarf over your mouth and nose so you inhale warm air.

If you enjoy team sports, try those that require short bursts of activity, such as

- Baseball
- Softball
- Volleyball
- Tennis
- Football
- Wrestling
- Short-term track and field events
- Golfing

Treatment

If your doctor determines you have exercise-induced asthma, you may be given inhaled medication to take before exercising. The most common medicine is a short-acting inhaled bronchodilator used fifteen minutes before exercise. If this treatment isn't sufficient, your doctor may consider giving you long-term control medicine to take daily.

Think about . . .
my favorite types of exercise

The type of exercise I enjoy most is_____.

This exercise can bring on
asthma symptoms.   ___YES ___NO

Another type of exercise I can try is_____.

I do a warm-up before
starting to exercise.   ___YES ___NO

I do a cool-down after exercising. ___YES ___NO

I've talked to my doctor about
asthma and exercise.   ___YES ___NO

> You should also warm up before
> exercising, and do a cool-down, including
> stretching and jogging, to prevent air in your
> lungs from changing temperature too quickly.
>   Avoid exercising when you have a cold or other
> respiratory infection, or when it's very cold
> outside. If your asthma is triggered by air
> pollution or pollen, avoid exercising outdoors
> when levels of these irritants are high.

"He wants to run and jump like any other kid—his asthma doesn't stop him. He won't quit—he just gets his inhaler and keeps going."

—RACHEL G., MOTHER OF AN EIGHT-YEAR-OLD WITH ASTHMA

Camp Catch Your Breath

We arrived at Jackson's Mill, West Virginia, that afternoon not knowing what to expect. We unloaded our suitcases, then my mom went to sign us in at the camp registration table while my grandmother took a reluctant look around.

After we were signed in, we headed into our cabin, picked out beds and made them. "You girls don't have to stay here, you can come home with us right now," my mother said as her eyes welled with tears. "We'll be okay, Mommy," my sister and I replied.

It was our first time at camp. Mandy was nine and I was eight. "Are you sure you'll be okay?" "Yes, Mommy."

So we headed outside. Mom kissed us good-bye and told us she loved us. We started to play with another one of the campers. Mom and Grandma stood by the cabin and watched us play, and the camp director came over and reassured them that we would be all right. So in tears, Mom and Grandma departed.

We were at Camp Catch Your Breath, a little camp held every year at Jackson's Mill for children with asthma. I had enjoyed myself so far, but a little while later I found myself sitting on my bed, a single tear streaming down my face. I missed my mom. But soon enough, I was having a blast with everyone in camp.

By the end of the week, I had had so much fun that I cried because I didn't want to leave. I had also learned so much that week. I found out that my asthma could not limit what I do, that I in fact had the control. I was better able to handle any scary situation with my asthma that arose and all that I owe to the wonderful people who took the time out of their summer to educate children about their asthma.

I returned to camp every year after that. To this day I attend Camp Catch Your Breath, but now as a counselor. Growing up through the program, I felt it was my responsibility to give back to a camp that gave me so much. It's not only something that I love to do, but it's an extremely fulfilling experience to know that you can make a difference in children's lives, by helping them to realize that they are in control of their life and their asthma, and that just because they have asthma doesn't mean that they can't do everything that every other "normal" kid can. They can achieve their dreams.

♥ *Jessica Rogerson*

Asthma in Children

Asthma is the leading chronic illness in children. Fortunately, most children with asthma have mild to moderate problems, and their breathing problems can be controlled with treatment at home. If your child is being kept awake at night, isn't able to participate in their favorite activities like ballet or soccer, or is missing school because of their asthma, then it's not under control—and you need to let your child's doctor know.

In young children, asthma symptoms may be missed. That's because wheezing isn't the only sign of asthma in children. Frequent coughing, inability to keep up with other children during play and unusual irritability also may be signs of asthma.

Children with frequent respiratory infections (such as pneumonia or bronchitis) should be checked by their doctor for asthma. A feeling of tightness in the chest and shortness of breath also can be signs of asthma.

TREATMENT

Your child's doctor will choose medication for your child based on his or her symptoms and test results. Children's asthma medications often are the same as those for adults, but doses are smaller. Children with asthma may need both a quick-relief inhaler if they feel an asthma attack coming on, and daily medication to control their asthma.

Your child's doctor may ask you to help your child use a peak flow meter to help keep their asthma under control. Measuring a child's lung function with a peak flow meter can be very helpful because it may be hard for a child to describe the symptoms.

You will need to take your child to the doctor for regular follow-up visits and make sure that your child uses the medication properly.

Your doctor may recommend a special device to help your child take asthma medication such as a spacer, which makes it easier for a child to use an inhaler, or nebulizer, which delivers medication in a mist that the child inhales. Your doctor will show you and your child how to take the medicine and use any special devices. If you are not completely sure how to use them, ask again!!

Treatment Tips

- If your child uses a bronchodilator inhaler to deal with asthma symptoms, he or she should begin to feel better within five to ten minutes.
- It usually takes one hour for liquid medicines to work. For pills and capsules, the time varies, so check with your doctor or pharmacist.
- Asthma medicines, including corticosteroids, are safe and highly effective if taken in the recommended doses. All medicines can be harmful if they are not taken properly.
- If your child experiences any side effects from asthma medication, call your doctor. If your doctor cannot be reached, reduce the dose by half, or skip the next dose. Do not stop the medicine completely. This may cause the asthma to get worse.
- Asthma medicine taken by mouth should never be taken on an empty stomach. If your child gets nauseous or vomits, try to give the medicine with some milk or food. Be sure to tell your doctor you are doing this because giving the medicine with food or milk can change its effectiveness.
- If the side effects, such as vomiting, do not go away, talk to your doctor about changing the dose or the type of medicine. Vomiting is an urgent danger sign.

- Asthma medicine needs to be adjusted if your child has symptoms (such as wheezing or coughing) with exercise, at rest, at night or early in the morning. Speak to your doctor about changing the dose or type of medicine.
- For "as needed" medicines, give them within five minutes after symptoms begin. It takes less medicine to stop an episode in the early phases of asthma rather than later on.
- If your doctor agrees, give the medicine at the first sign of a cold or influenza even if you don't hear wheezing or coughing. Continue giving medicine until all signs of the cold or influenza are gone.
- Your child's doctor may prescribe medicine to be taken daily to prevent asthma even if your child does not have symptoms. The medicines reduce airway swelling and make it less likely that another episode will occur.

Think about . . .
my child's asthma

I would like help understanding

_____How my child should use the inhaler

_____How my child should use the peak flow
meter

_____How my child should use the spacer

_____How my child should use the nebulizer

Other questions I have: _____

_____

_____

_____

Think about . . .
my child's asthma symptoms

___ My child coughs, wheezes, has chest tightness or shortness of breath.

___ Colds go right to my child's chest and last much longer than other siblings.

___ My child coughs or wheezes with exercise, play and laughter or during temper tantrums.

___ We have a family history of asthma or allergies.

___ My child misses school because of asthma.

___ Coughing or wheezing keeps me and my child up at night.

My child's asthma triggers are _____

_____

_____

_____

This is how often my child's symptoms happen, and how bad they are:

_____

_____

_____

Take this checklist to your child's next doctor appointment and discuss it with the doctor.

*"I want all kids with asthma to know that when
you take care of yourself and your asthma, you can
still run and have fun!"*

—SCOTT H., AGE TWELVE

Running on Asthma

Our family doesn't think of asthma as a bad
thing; it's just a fact of life in our house. Both my
sons have asthma; my youngest son, Sydney, has
been a severe asthmatic since he was three months
old. His older brother, Bradley, has asthma, too, but
not as severe. Sure, they'd rather not have it, but
they do. I have always explained to them that having asthma is like having blue or brown eyes; it is
just part of who they are.

I've discussed with both boys that kids can die
from asthma and that is why they have to always
take their medication correctly. They both know the
medications that they have to take and the schedule
for taking them. They also know to pretreat before
playing too hard (sports, tag, running around).

Sydney is the most coordinated, athletic child I
have ever seen. It can be difficult to balance his

athletic gifts with his asthma. He started running before he was nine months old and I was always trying to slow him down for fear of another asthma attack. Sydney would run as fast as he could, stop suddenly and drop to the ground, catch his breath, and then get up and run some more.

One day I was talking with his physician about the balance between running and asthma. He told me that I have to let Sydney be a "normal" child. He has to be able to follow his dreams; we just have to do it with an inhaler in hand. I finally relented and allowed Sydney to join a baseball team when he was four years old. I was so scared, but I just gave him his medication before the start of the game and held his rescue meds in my hand during all the games.

I had never seen my son so happy. He was doing what he loved . . . playing baseball with the other kids on a team. It has been a year since Sydney first played on a baseball team and since then he has taken ice skating lessons, joined a sports club at school, played street hockey with his big brother and cannot wait to join a team again soon.

It is still hard to let him go, but I know that I have to. More important, he feels he can do anything . . . and he can!

♥ *Shari Davis Gonzales*

Coping with Your Child's Asthma

Finding out your child has asthma can produce a range of emotions. You may be relieved to know what's been causing your child distress. Or you might feel overwhelmed thinking that you'll be dealing with a long-term condition, and you wonder how you'll manage if your child has an asthma attack. It's natural to worry, but with time, and experience, you'll feel more confident about dealing with asthma.

Many children handle the news that they have asthma better than their parents do. It's important to keep a positive attitude. Don't let your concern overshadow your child's growing independence. Hovering over children will not help them.

However, there may be times when you have to make decisions that affect their health—such as deciding that your child can't go to a friend's house because their cat can trigger your child's asthma. Simply say no, tell your child why, and don't dwell on it. Getting stuck in guilt won't help your child— or you.

Help children take responsibility for their asthma as they get older. They'll gain pride and self-confidence when they master the day-to-day tasks involved in caring for their asthma. Praise them as they take on more responsibility, and acknowledge that it can be scary for you to let go a little bit. But remember, they will need to learn to care for themselves as they grow.

Preschoolers can:

- Help with peak flow monitoring with close parental supervision.
- Start to find words to describe their symptoms.

School-age children can:

- Perform peak flow monitoring and take medications with supervision.
- Tell parents when they feel an early onset of asthma symptoms.
- Be allowed to play and participate in sports.

Pre-teens can:

- Understand the consequences of failing to manage asthma.
- Have more independence in taking medication, peak flow monitoring and following their asthma action plan.

Some coping tips for parents of children with asthma:

- It's important to remember that with proper medical care, your child with asthma *can* have a normal childhood.

- Realize the impact that your child's asthma is having on his or her siblings. Schedule some one-on-one time with your nonasthmatic children. Plan a special activity, or cook their favorite meal once in awhile—it's a way of showing them that they're special too.
- Don't downplay the stress that dealing with your child's asthma causes. You're coping with fears of your child's illness, visiting the doctor and managing your child's medication regimen. You need to get enough sleep and eat nutritiously. Otherwise, you won't have enough energy for yourself or your family.
- Get sources of support—friends, family and local support groups for parents of children with asthma. Contact local groups such as the American Lung Association, Allergy and Asthma Network/Mothers of Asthmatics and the Allergy and Asthma Foundation of America to find out what information and help they can offer you.
- Read as much as you can about asthma—the more you know, the easier it will be for you to deal with your child's health in a confident and calm manner.

READER/CUSTOMER CARE SURVEY

CEAG

We care about your opinions! Please take a moment to fill out our online Reader Survey at **http://survey.hcibooks.com.** As a **"THANK YOU"** you will receive a **VALUABLE INSTANT COUPON** towards future book purchases as well as a **SPECIAL GIFT** available only online! Or, you may mail this card back to us and we will send you a copy of our exciting catalog with your valuable coupon inside.

First Name _____ MI. _____ Last Name _____

Address _____ City _____

State _____ Zip _____ Email _____

1. Gender
- ☐ Female
- ☐ Male

2. Age
- ☐ 8 or younger
- ☐ 9-12
- ☐ 13-16
- ☐ 17-20
- ☐ 21-30
- ☐ 31+

3. Did you receive this book as a gift?
- ☐ Yes
- ☐ No

4. Annual Household Income
- ☐ under $25,000
- ☐ $25,000 - $34,999
- ☐ $35,000 - $49,999
- ☐ $50,000 - $74,999
- ☐ over $75,000

5. What are the ages of the children living in your house?
- ☐ 0 - 14
- ☐ 15+

6. Marital Status
- ☐ Single
- ☐ Married
- ☐ Divorced
- ☐ Widowed

Comments
_____
_____
_____
_____
_____

Do you have your own Chicken Soup story that you would like to send us?
Please submit at: **www.chickensoup.com**

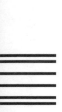

BUSINESS REPLY MAIL
FIRST-CLASS MAIL PERMIT NO 45 DEERFIELD BEACH, FL

POSTAGE WILL BE PAID BY ADDRESSEE

Chicken Soup for the Soul®
Healthy Living Series
3201 SW 15th Street
Deerfield Beach FL 33442-9875

Think about . . .
how I feel about my child's asthma

My concerns about my child's asthma are

_____

_____

_____

A time when I wasn't sure what to do about my
child's asthma was _____

_____

_____

_____

I'd like to improve the way I handle my child's
asthma by _____

_____

_____

"I can see his symptoms before
he can even feel them."

—BARBARA BEROFF, MOTHER OF A TEN-YEAR-OLD SON WITH ASTHMA

Like Mother, Like Son

I left the pediatrician's office with an infant carrier in one hand and a brand new nebulizer in the other. I had presented a brave face in the doctor's office, but tears welled up as I walked to my car. My beautiful, angelic baby boy was what I had prayed he wouldn't be—a wheezer. I secured the baby in the car and sat in the driver's seat and cried. Like me, my baby was destined for a life of "can'ts"— can't spend the night with a friend with a pet, can't run barefoot through a grassy field, can't leave home without an inhaler.

My son's medication regimen was new to me. As we began his treatment plan, which included a daily maintenance drug, I learned more about new medications and how far science has come to control asthma symptoms. Control asthma? I thought you just rolled with the punches—or rather the coughs and wheezes. I was using a store-bought inhaler and used it when I needed it, which was a lot more than the directions on the package recommended.

A few months later, two back-to-back asthma attacks sent me to the emergency room, sweating and in danger. The physician treated me and said, "It would be really senseless for you to die of an asthma attack. Asthma is so treatable. But left untreated, there is no resuscitating the overworked lungs." I thought of my husband and baby waiting for me at home. *Okay, Lord, I understand now. I have to plan to be around for a long time, to see my children grow up and have children of their own. I have to lead by example for my son about how to live with asthma. It is up to me.*

I went home and called a specialist. After meeting with him, all my excuses fell away. New mom, too tired, too busy—I had no good excuse for not taking charge of my health.

Today, my son and I each take a daily maintenance drug. I have done my best to avoid our "triggers" and am prepared to treat symptoms quickly. My son is young enough that I pray that he will outgrow his asthma. But if he doesn't, that's okay. We can live, and live well, with asthma.

♥ *Shawn Scott McSwain*

How to Head Off
a Child's Asthma Attack

Every child with asthma has a built-in early warning system that signals when an asthma attack is impending. Even if your child is not old enough to tell you how they feel, you can learn to look for the signs before the symptoms get bad.

WARNING SIGNS

- Cough
- Unusual paleness or sweating
- Anxious or scared look
- Flared nostrils when the child tries to get some air
- Pursed lips breathing
- Fast breathing
- Vomiting
- Hunched-over body posture; the child can't stand or sit straight and can't relax
- Restlessness during sleep
- Fatigue that isn't related to working or playing hard
- The notch just above the child's Adam's apple sinks in as they breathe in
- Spaces between the ribs sink in when the child breathes in

WHAT TO LISTEN FOR

- Coughing when the child has no cold
- Clearing of the throat a lot
- Irregular breathing
- Wheezing, however light
- Noisy, difficult breathing

HOW TO LISTEN

Put your ear to the child's back and your hand on his or her chest. You'll feel the chest go up as the child inhales, drawing in air, and you'll feel the chest go down as the child exhales, releasing air.

- Listen for squeaking or any unusual noises. They may mean asthma, bronchitis or a chest infection. Only a doctor can tell for sure, so regard any noisy breathing as a signal that help may be necessary.
- If the child is having symptoms and there are no chest sounds, call your doctor immediately.

WHAT TO DO IMMEDIATELY

Reassure the child by your tone of voice, your attitude of being able to manage, your confidence. All those qualities are catching. Your child will take cues from you and relax.

- If the doctor has recommended a medicine when signals appear, use it. (Don't give the child a special dose unless the doctor said to).

- Encourage normal fluid intake. Drinking too much may actually hurt, not help.

EMERGENCY SIGNS

Call your doctor or get emergency medical care if your child exhibits any of these signs.

- Wheeze, cough or shortness of breath gets worse, even after the medicine has been given time to work. Most inhaled bronchodilator medications produce an effect within five to ten minutes. Discuss the time your medicines take to work with your child's doctor.
- Child has a hard time breathing. Signs of this are:
  — Chest and neck are pulled or sucked in with each breath.
  — Struggling to breathe.
  — Child has trouble walking or talking, stops playing and cannot start again.
  — Peak flow rate gets lower or does not improve after treatment with bronchodilators or drops to 50 percent or less of your child's personal best.
  — Lips or fingernails are gray or blue. If this happens, GO TO THE DOCTOR OR EMERGENCY ROOM RIGHT AWAY!

Think about . . .
my child's asthma action checklist

__ I know the signs of a possible asthma attack in my child.

__ I know what peak flow readings signal a possible attack.

__ I know what medications to use if my child shows signs of breathing trouble.

__ I know how to use the medications.

__ I know where the medications are kept.

__ I know where my child's asthma action plan is.

__ I have the phone number of my child's doctor posted where it is easily seen.

__ I know the name and location of the nearest hospital.

God Knew What I Could Handle

My son Kevin was born premature 12 years ago. I had him when I was 30 weeks into my pregnancy. We had many obstacles to overcome. I never imagined that asthma would be my biggest one.

Kevin was diagnosed with asthma nine years ago. I had no idea that asthma would have such an impact on our lives. I am a divorced mother of three. My other children are 20 and 14. Asthma has affected all of our lives tremendously.

Asthma requires many sacrifices. Each day I pack medicines and a nebulizer machine to go to school with Kevin. When we want to go for an outing, I have to be totally aware of weather and environmental surroundings. When I visit other people, I have to make sure that they don't have pets and no one in the home smokes. Vacations require a lot of preparation. I have to make sure that I inform the doctor. I always have to know where the closest hospital is.

I used to feel that I was being punished because

of the endless nights that I spend awake, the hours that I have to worry about him during the day and the amount of days that I have to miss from my job, And I can't give my other two children the same amount of attention that they deserve.

Then I realized I wasn't being punished.

I feel special because I was chosen to have a child with asthma. It takes a special parent to handle all the obstacles that come along with asthma. I now feel privileged, because God knew what I could handle. When I see Kevin smile or he hugs me I know that I was chosen.

Kevin still misses about 25 days a year from school because of asthma (less than half the number of days he used to miss) and has remained on the honor roll for the last seven years. When he was nine, Kevin was able to play in the snow for the first time in his life. Even more exciting was the news we just received that Kevin is now well enough to join the basketball team. He has achieved his lifelong dream.

♥ *Renee Hall-Freeman*

Asthma at School

The best way for you to be sure that your child's asthma will be well controlled during school is to communicate with your child's teacher, school nurse and physical education teacher. Here's what you'll need to do:

- **Write down your child's asthma and allergy triggers** (such as exercise, pet dander or specific foods). Give the list to teachers, coaches, nurses and other grownups who will be in charge of your child during the school day.
- **Give the school staff a written list of your child's medications.** Include dosages and instructions about when the medications should be taken.
- **Give the nurse emergency medications** along with written instructions for how to respond to an asthma attack or allergic reaction.
- **Provide a list of emergency phone numbers** including your child's doctor.
- **Talk to the school staff about your child's asthma warning signs.**

HOW ASTHMA-FRIENDLY IS YOUR SCHOOL?
A CHECKLIST

Children with asthma need proper support at school to keep their asthma under control and be

fully active. Use the questions below to find out
how well your child's school helps children with
asthma.

                                          YES   NO

1. Is your school free of tobacco
   smoke at all times, including
   during school-sponsored events?   ____   ____

2. Does the school maintain good
   indoor air quality? Does it
   reduce or eliminate allergens
   and irritants that can make
   asthma worse? Check if any of
   the following are present: ____   ____
   ___Cockroaches
   ___Dust mites (commonly
      found in humid climates
      in pillows, carpets, upholstery
      and stuffed toys)
   ___Mold
   ___Pets with fur or feathers
   ___Strong odors or fumes from
      art and craft supplies, pesticides,
      paint, perfumes, air fresheners
      and cleaning chemicals

3. Is there a school nurse in your
   school all day, every day? If not, ____   ____
   is a nurse regularly available to
   help the school write plans and

	YES	NO

give the school guidance on
medicines, physical education,
and field trips for students
with asthma? ___ ___

4. Can children take medicines at
school as recommended by their
doctor and parents? May children ___ ___
carry their own asthma medicines? ___ ___

5. Does your school have a written,
individualized emergency plan for
each child in case of a severe
asthma episode (attack)? Does the ___ ___
plan make clear what action to
take? Whom to call? When to call? ___ ___

6. Does someone teach school staff
about asthma, asthma management
plans and asthma medicines? ___ ___
Does someone teach all students
about asthma and how to help a
classmate who has it? ___ ___

7. Do students have good options
for fully and safely participating
in physical education class and
recess? (For example, do students ___ ___
have access to their medicine
before exercise? Can they choose ___ ___
modified or alternative activities
when medically necessary?) ___ ___

If the answer to any question is "no," your child may face obstacles to good asthma control at school. Talk to the principal and school nurse about making your child's school more asthma-friendly. If you need help, contact one of the organizations listed in the Resources section of this book.

"Anyone with asthma knows the fear of not being
able to breathe—it's the rest of the world that
needs to understand."

—DEBRA W., MOTHER OF TEEN WITH ASTHMA

Asthma at Sixteen

My name is Jessica and I was diagnosed with asthma at the age of six. Here I am now at the ripe age of 16, 10 years later looking back at the ups and downs I've been through growing up with asthma.

Now to someone who doesn't have asthma nor has any knowledge of the disease, this probably would seem like some exaggeration and that asthma is just a ploy for attention or as a gym teacher once put it, "just an excuse," but asthma is a problem that affects millions of children every day.

Today, people are more understanding now that asthma is, in fact, seen as a serious issue, and that it does make seemingly simple activities difficult for a child, such as a game of tag with friends or going out in winter to build a snowman.

I've realized as I've gotten older that it's become

sort of a joke with my friends. They sort of kid about it or call me "wheezer" every once in a while. But when it comes down to it, any time I get out of breath or begin to have a problem with my asthma around my friends, they are always the first to notice and offer help: "Are you all right? Do you have your inhaler with you?"

With all the knowledge I have gained, I am in better control of my asthma, but sometimes it gets the best of me and I panic. But I am lucky to be surrounded by such caring and understanding individuals.

Whenever I feel like my asthma is winning, I just remind myself that I am in control of my asthma and that I can achieve anything I set my mind to. My asthma can't stop me from achieving my dreams.

♥ *Jessica Lynn Blazier*

Asthma Throughout Your Life

There are certain times in a person's life that asthma presents special challenges: the teen years, during pregnancy, and later in life.

TEENS AND ASTHMA

The teenage years can be the worst time to feel different. And that's just how asthma can make teens feel. They may feel uncomfortable having to take medicine or using an inhaler or peak flow meter in front of friends.

Teens with asthma may encounter tough situations—deciding whether to decline an invitation to the house of a friend who has pets that can trigger an asthma attack, or having to sit out a team practice on a day when asthma symptoms are flaring up.

Some teens with asthma may end up avoiding physical activity altogether for fear of having an attack in front of others. Others may use asthma as an excuse to get out of gym class or other activities they don't want to do. What's especially dangerous is when teens forget—or refuse—to take their asthma medicine to prevent or control breathing problems. That can lead to a trip to the hospital if a teen's asthma gets out of control.

The goals for teens with asthma are to

- Understand their disease
- Have a simple asthma action plan
- Feel in control of their lives
- Realize that asthma doesn't define who they are or limit them

If you're a parent of a teen with asthma, it's important to realize that asthma may affect your child's self-esteem. You need to be aware of the possibility that your teen is minimizing asthma symptoms or avoiding taking asthma medication in order to appear just like his or her friends.

Being a parent is never easy, but parenting a teen with asthma has its own special challenges—trying to make sure teens are following their asthma action plan, while giving them the independence to make decisions about their own health.

Some parents of teens with asthma may find it's useful to make a contract with their teens that outlines an asthma management plan and offers rewards and consequences.

You are more likely to avoid confrontations about your teen's asthma if you talk with your teen about what he or she can do to take control of their breathing. Think about what you've been saying—have you been heavy on restrictions and limits, emphasizing what your teen can't do because of asthma?

Instead, accentuate the positive—talk about what your teen can do. Give as much responsibility as you think your teen can handle. Emphasize that now that your teen is older and more independent, it's time to be more responsible for his or her own health. Talk to teens about what can happen if their asthma isn't managed properly and remind them that controlling their asthma will allow them to do the activities they enjoy. Then trust your teen to take medicine at the right time, in the right way. He or she is sure to appreciate your confidence in his or her ability to manage his or her own health.

Offer support and encouragement by

- Allowing your teen to meet with the doctor alone. This will encourage your teen to become more involved in his or her own asthma care.
- Encouraging your teen to meet other teens with asthma so they can offer one another support.

Think about . . .
your teen's asthma

My teenager's feelings about asthma are _____
_____
_____
_____

Problems I've encountered in trying to help my teen manage asthma are _____
_____
_____
_____

Something that's worked in helping my teen deal with asthma is _____
_____
_____
_____

I wish my teenager with asthma would_____
_____
_____
_____

Asthma and Pregnancy

If you're pregnant and have asthma, it's especially important for you to stick to your asthma action plan—for the sake of your health as well as your baby's.

It's understandable that a woman with asthma may wonder whether it's okay to take medicine. Studies have shown that most inhaled asthma medications are safe for pregnant women. If you take asthma pills, talk to your doctor about whether you can switch to another medication during your pregnancy.

The good news is that women whose asthma is well controlled during pregnancy have a very good chance of having a normal pregnancy and a healthy baby. Uncontrolled asthma, on the other hand, can lead to a decrease in the amount of oxygen in the mother's blood, which means a decrease in oxygen for the fetus. This can affect fetal growth, because the fetus needs a constant supply of oxygen for normal growth. Uncontrolled asthma can lead to premature birth and a baby with low birth weight.

As soon as you find out you're pregnant, talk with your doctor about your asthma medications and whether they are appropriate and safe to use during pregnancy.

Important facts about asthma and pregnancy include:

- Some women find their asthma gets better during pregnancy, some find it gets worse and others find it stays the same. If your asthma changes, your doctor will adjust your medicine as needed.
- Asthma tends to get worse in the late second and early third trimester of pregnancy. If your asthma is well controlled during pregnancy, you are very unlikely to have asthma troubles during labor and delivery.
- Most women with asthma can perform Lamaze breathing techniques without any trouble.
- Talk to your doctor about getting a flu shot. Influenza is especially dangerous for people with asthma.
- If you smoke, now's the time to quit! Smoking may make your asthma worse, and it directly affects the health of your growing baby. Also avoid being around other people's smoke— secondhand smoke can trigger your asthma and affect your baby, too.

OLDER ADULTS AND ASTHMA

Developing asthma in adulthood can be a big surprise. Some adults who develop asthma remember having had breathing problems as children, which went away, but came back later in life. Others develop asthma for the first time when they are older.

Sometimes an older person can have asthmalike symptoms such as wheezing that actually are the signs of another lung disease. Other lung diseases that cause similar problems are bronchitis and emphysema, especially in people who smoke. Heart disease can also cause breathing problems.

DRUG INTERACTIONS

If you're an older adult with asthma, there's a good chance you're taking medication for other health conditions as well. Some drugs may cause problems for people with asthma. Tell your doctor what medicines you are taking for other health problems. Don't forget to include alternative medicines and vitamin supplements. And remind your doctor about your asthma every time you get a new prescription. Keep an up-to-date list of all the medicines you take. Carry the list with you.

Drugs that may affect asthma include

- **Blood pressure and heart drugs.** Some people with asthma find that their asthma gets worse when they take certain blood pressure drugs such as beta-adrenergic blockers (such as propranolol, nadolol and timolol), or ACE inhibitors.

- **Pain relievers.** Some people with asthma may have breathing problems if they take aspirin, acetaminophen, ibuprofen or naproxen. Such drugs include many drugstore cold remedies and pain remedies.

TREATMENT TIPS

- If you're taking medications for several different conditions, work with your doctor to simplify your medication program as much as possible. Perhaps you can combine medications or use alternate ones that will have the same desired effect.
- Be sure your asthma action plan is written down, and give a copy to someone else—a family member, friend or neighbor.
- If you're having trouble using an inhaler because of arthritis, tell your doctor. If you don't use the inhaler correctly, you're not getting the correct dose. Ask your doctor whether you can use a breath-controlled inhaler, or a special device for inhalers for people with arthritis.
- Some asthma medications increase heart rate. If you feel an increased heart rate, be sure to tell your doctor.
- If you're taking oral steroids, you'll need regular checkups so your doctor can monitor you

for any signs of diabetes, hypertension, glau-
coma, cataracts and osteoporosis.

- Ask your doctor about getting an annual flu
  shot and a pneumonia shot (which may be
  given every five years to adults 65 and older).

Think about . . .
my doctor's visit checklist

__ Tell my doctor if I've had any change in asthma symptoms since my last visit.

__ Get written instructions on all my asthma medicines—how often to take and what dose.

__ Get written instructions on what to do when my asthma symptoms get worse.

__ Ask the doctor to show me how to properly use my inhaler and/or spacer device.

__ Ask for a peak flow meter and instructions on how to use it to monitor my lung function.

__ Bring medications and peak flow records with me to each visit.

__ Tell my doctor if I've gotten any new prescriptions from any of my other doctors since my last visit.

__ Tell my doctor if I've had to go to the emergency room since my last visit.

My Asthma Friend

I was just over 40 when I was first told that the breathlessness I had been experiencing was asthma. At first, it didn't really strike me as anything too serious. I would take my two different inhalers and I would be fine.

The trouble started when my doctor arranged for me to attend his asthma clinic at our local county hospital. As I walked into the waiting area, there didn't seem to be anyone there under 70 years of age.

I sat there looking around me, thinking everyone looked old and ill. There was frequent coughing, wheezing and I suddenly saw my future before me and was horrified. I began to realize that asthma was something to be taken seriously.

Following that visit, I read up on the different kinds of asthma and the treatments. I found out that, fortunately, my asthma was not too serious and mainly it was a question of getting it under control with the correct medication.

I went to two more of the clinics and hated each

one. At the second one, one of the older gentlemen introduced himself as Ben and tried to make conversation with me. He seemed to have trouble breathing and it was difficult to follow what he was saying. I had little to say to poor Ben; all I wanted was not to end up like him. I was still the youngest person there and after my third visit, I told my doctor I was not going to any further sessions.

For a few months, I had my medication adjusted here and there and was getting on fine. Then, I got a terrible head cold; it lasted for two weeks and went from my head into my chest. I developed a bad wheezy cough that I had never really had before and my asthma was awful. I had to inhale four or five times to get any kind of relief.

I stayed out of work, but one day my husband was working out of town and, feeling a little better, I went into town for some shopping. I was coming out of a shop when I started to cough. I couldn't stop and my wheezing got so bad that I remember collapsing on to the sidewalk gasping for breath, my inhaler useless in my hand. I heard people say, "Call an ambulance, she is choking. . . ."

That was when a calm voice said, "No, an ambulance will take too long, she's having an asthma attack. Help her over to my car, I'll drive her to a doctor." Someone argued and the man said, "I am an asthmatic, she needs to get to a nebulizer as soon as possible. The doctor's office is not far away."

I remember getting into the car, still trying to breathe and in a state of panic. He told me, "Calm down, breathe slowly, let your inhaler do the work."

I did as he said and he drove me the five minutes to the doctor's office. As soon as we got there, he rushed in and people came out to help me. I was soon attached to the nebulizer, the mask over my face and starting to breathe again. The doctor explained that my asthma was pretty well controlled but that getting a really bad chest cold may always be more of a problem, and might require additional medication.

"You were lucky your friend was there and had the sense to bring you straight in to the nebulizer. Waiting for an ambulance would not have been a good idea," he said. "He said you panicked a little. The reason for going to the asthma clinic was to help you cope with that kind of situation."

I nodded. "I'm sorry, I just felt uncomfortable at the clinic. You said my friend—I was so distressed, I don't really know who the gentleman was."

"His name is Ben Patterson. You probably met him at the asthma clinic. He is a wonderful old gentleman. He has bad asthma but never lets it get in his way, still takes long walks, goes off abroad on vacation. He is so eager to help people who are first diagnosed and may think that their world has come to an end. Wasn't he at the clinic when you were there?" he asked me. "Yes, I think he was," I said, not willing to admit I had brushed aside the help of this man who had probably saved my life.

I cried when I told my husband about it later and said, "I must find out where he lives and go and thank him," I said. "Why don't you thank him by going along to the next clinic and listening to what he has to say?" Eric suggested.

I did exactly that. I apologized for how I had responded the first time and thanked him for saving my life. Ben and I became firm friends; he had traveled all over the world and had endless tales to tell of his adventures. He was one of the most interesting people I had ever met and he gave me so much good advice about my asthma. "Accept that you have it, get it under control and get on with your life. If you have to make adjustments around it, then do so, but don't let it have the upper hand in what you can and cannot do, you decide!"

When Ben passed away, some years ago now, there were so many people like me at his funeral. I had met most of them through Ben, and Eric laughingly refers to them as "Your asthma friends." We still talk about Ben and try to pass on to others what this lovely man taught us.

♥ *Joyce Stark*

Traveling with Asthma

People with asthma and their families love vacation time just as much as anybody else. But having asthma means needing some extra preparation before going on a trip.

Here are some tips for having a vacation where you can breathe easy:

MEDICATIONS

- Bring your asthma action plan with you!
- Bring a list of medications that includes the prescription refill number, the name and phone number of the doctor who prescribed it, and the dosage (all this information should be on the medicine's original label).
- Pack not only the amount of medicine you think you'll need, but also a backup quantity just in case you end up staying longer or need extra for any reason. Pack your medication in your carry-on luggage just in case your checked luggage gets lost.
- If you have an emergency epinephrine injection kit for allergic reactions, bring it with you.

EQUIPMENT

- Bring your peak flow meter along with the chart to record results.

- If you use a nebulizer, bring it along. Portable nebulizers are available that can be plugged into the cigarette lighter in a car.
- If you are traveling abroad, make sure you have an electrical current converter for the nebulizer.
- If your asthma is triggered by dust mites, you may want to bring your own allergy-proof pillow or mattress cover.
- If you'll be by yourself in unfamiliar surroundings, consider wearing a medical alert-type necklace or bracelet.

HEALTH INSURANCE

- Ask your doctor for recommendations for an asthma specialist at your destination, or contact the local state medical society at your vacation spot for recommendations.
- Call your health insurance company to find out what they will cover in another state or country, and whether your plan will cover doctor and hospital visits where you are going.

OTHER TRAVEL TIPS

- Ask for a smoke-free hotel room.
- If you're traveling by car, run the air conditioner or heater, with the windows open, for at least ten minutes to reduce mold and dust mites in the car.

If your asthma is affected by pollen or pollution, travel with the car windows closed and the air conditioner on.

While all airplanes within the United States are smoke-free, that's not true for international travel. Ask for a smoke-free flight, or if that's not available, ask for a seat that's as far away as possible from the smoking section.

If you'll be staying with friends or family, explain your or your child's asthma triggers. It may not be a good idea to stay with a family with pets, or with a smoker unless that person agrees to smoke outside during your stay.

If you're camping, be aware that cold air and wood fires may trigger asthma.

Think about . . .
planning my trip

For my next trip I'd love to travel to _____

_____

_____

_____

I'll need to find out these things about potential asthma triggers at my destination: _____

_____

_____

_____

Potential problems that might arise from traveling to this place are _____

_____

_____

_____

Possible solutions are_____

_____

_____

_____

"With changes in my medication and
asthma management, I've been able to
train to run a marathon."

—CHRIS T., SCHOOL NURSE

I'm Breathing!

Breathing—how often I took it for granted when I was young. Sure, I had frequent colds and wheezing breaths, but I never knew that I had asthma. At the age of 44, I had my first life-threatening asthma attack. I resisted being put on prednisone, because I didn't want to gain weight. I just would not believe that I could die. I was revived on the floor of my physician's office with four alarmed doctors hovering over me. It took four shots of prednisone to save my life and three weeks of high doses of oral prednisone. I don't know which was worse, almost dying or the lingering weeks of recovery.

In the last 15 years, I have discovered just how precious I am, especially to my family. I have been blessed with the devotion of my daughters, as they keep their vigilant watch over me when I am desperately ill. They have shared their thoughts and dreams with me and have made me laugh and cry.

My asthma has given me something else very precious. It has given me time. Time—the one rare ingredient that the rest of the world can't seem to find. If only there were more hours to the day, days to the week, weeks to the year, then there would be enough time. The more hurried the world becomes, the less time it can capture. I am blessed. I have plenty of time. I can walk slowly on the good days, and I can see more of what I missed when I didn't take the time. I can write the things that are nearest and dearest to my heart.

The most remarkable gift I have received, however, is an inner peace. I no longer rush through the good things in life. I seize the opportunity to watch the blazing sunset from beginning to end. I meet the rosy dawn in the mountains where I live, with a song in my heart as the sun chases away the ribbons of the night. I am thankful for every breath, knowing that my Creator holds each one in His hand. I see the love in my husband's eyes when he looks at me, knowing within those dark green depths that he has never looked upon anyone so lovely.

There are new treatments for asthma, and I am on an aggressive regimen. In 1994, my pulmonologist promised me that within 10 years there would be new drugs approved that would be nothing short of miraculous. I didn't believe her, yet it has become a reality for me. My serious asthma attacks are now fewer and farther apart. Thankfully, they are shorter and less life-threatening. I make certain to keep up with the latest treatments, and I keep a good working relationship with my doctor, based on mutual respect and trust.

At 59, I am in charge of my asthma, instead of my asthma being in charge of me. Asthma has given me many things. It has given me strength and determination, so that I will never let it conquer my spirit. I am thankful for each new day. I have faith. I have hope. I have love. I am precious. Life is beautiful, because I'm breathing!

♥ *Jaye Lewis*

Breathing Easier

By following all the steps outlined in this book and working closely with your doctor, you should be well on your way to breathing easier. You know your asthma, or your child's asthma, is under control if you can say

__I don't cough.

__I don't have shortness of breath or rapid breathing, wheezing or chest tightness.

__I don't wake up at night because of asthma symptoms.

__I can engage in normal activities including play, sports and exercise.

__My child isn't absent from school or activities because of asthma.

__I'm not missing any time from work because of asthma.

__I haven't had any asthma episodes lately that require a visit to the doctor or emergency room.

__My lung function is normal or near normal.

__I only need my reliever medication less than twice a week.

One thing I've always wanted to do but never have because of asthma is _____

_____

Now that you have a plan to keep your asthma under control, there's no excuse. Now you have it in writing, it's up to you to make it happen. Enjoy!

Resources

Allergy and Asthma Network—Mothers of Asthmatics, Inc.
2751 Prosperity Avenue, Suite 150, Fairfax, VA 22031 (1-800-878-4403; 703-385-4403, Fax: 703-573-7794) Newsletter: The MA Report *http://www.aanma.org/*

American Academy of Allergy, Asthma & Immunology
611 East Wells St., Milwaukee, WI 53202 (1-800-822-2762; 414-272-6071) *http://www.aaaai.org/*

American College of Allergy, Asthma and Immunology.
85 W. Algonquin Rd., Suite 550, Arlington Heights, IL 60005 (847-427-1200) *http://www.acaai.org/*

American Lung Association
For your local chapter or a respiratory therapist: 1-800-LUNG-USA. National Headquarters: 61 Broadway, 6th floor, New York, NY 10006 (212-315-8700) *http://www.lungusa.org/*

Asthma and Allergy Foundation of America
1233 20th St. NW, Ste. 402, Washington, DC 20036 (1-800-7ASTHMA; 202-466-7643, Fax: 202-466-8940) Newsletter: *The Asthma and Allergy Advance http://www.aafa.org/*

Centers for Disease Control and Prevention
To learn more about asthma, visit *www.cdc.gov/asthma.*

Environmental Protection Agency (EPA)
To learn more about controlling indoor asthma triggers, visit *www.epa.gov/asthma*. Call the EPA's Indoor Air Quality Information Line at 1-800-438-4318 to order free materials about indoor asthma triggers. To learn more about the Air Quality Index (AQI), visit *www.epa.gov/airnow*.

National Heart, Lung, and Blood Institute Information Center, National Institutes of Health
PO Box 30105, Bethesda, MD 20824-0105 (301-592-8573) *http://www.nhlbi.nih.gov/*

National Jewish Medical and Research Center
1400 Jackson St., Denver, CO 80206 (303-388-4461) *www.NationalJewish.org/*

Lung Line. 1-800-222-LUNG.
Talk to a nurse and request printed information be sent to you. Library Information Pathfinder on the Web and in the Library; a multilevel approach to information access from the Gerald Tucker Memorial Medical Library.

Supporting Organization

✝ **AMERICAN LUNG ASSOCIATION.**

The American Lung Association is the oldest voluntary health organization in the United States, with a national office and constituent associations around the country. It works to prevent lung disease and promote lung health. Lung diseases and breathing problems are the primary causes of infant deaths in the United States today, and asthma is the leading serious chronic childhood illness. Smoking remains the nation's number one preventable cause of death. Lung disease death rates continue to increase while other major causes of death have declined.

The American Lung Association has long funded research to discover the causes and seek improved treatments for those suffering with lung disease. They are the foremost defender of the Clean Air Act and laws that protect citizens from secondhand smoke. The Lung Association teaches children the dangers of tobacco use and helps teenage and adult smokers overcome tobacco addiction. They help children and adults living with lung disease to improve their quality of life. With the generous support of the American public, the American Lung Association is *"Improving life, one breath at a time."*

For more information about the American Lung Association or to support the work they do, call 1-800-LUNG-USA, or visit the Web site at *http://www.lungusa.org.*

Who Is Jack Canfield, Cocreator of *Chicken Soup for the Soul*?

Jack Canfield is one of America's leading experts in the development of human potential and personal effectiveness. He is both a dynamic, entertaining speaker and a highly sought-after trainer. Jack has a wonderful ability to inform and inspire audiences toward increased levels of self-esteem and peak performance. He has coauthored numerous books, including *Dare to Win, The Aladdin Factor, 100 Ways to Build Self-Concept in the Classroom, Heart at Work* and *The Power of Focus*. His latest book is *The Success Principles*.

www.jackcanfield.com

Who Is Mark Victor Hansen, Cocreator of *Chicken Soup for the Soul*?

In the area of human potential, no one is more respected than **Mark Victor Hansen**. For more than 30 years, Mark has focused solely on helping people from all walks of life reshape their personal vision of what's possible. His powerful messages of possibility, opportunity and action have created powerful change in thousands of organizations and millions of individuals nationwide. He is a prolific writer of bestselling books such as *The One Minute Millionaire, The Power of Focus, The Aladdin Factor,* and *Dare to Win*.

www.markvictorhansen.com

Who Is Norman H. Edelman, M.D.?

Norman H. Edelman, M.D., is vice president for Health Sciences and professor of medicine at SUNY Stony Brook University. He is also the chief medical officer for the American Lung Association.

Dr. Edelman is a member of the Association of Physicians, American Society for Clinical Investigation, American Federation for Clinical Research and the American Thoracic Society. In January of 1990, he was appointed to membership to the National Commission on Sleep Disorders Research. He is a fellow of the American College of Physicians and the American College of Chest Physicians.

A former member of the Editorial Boards for the Journal of Applied Physiology and the American Review of Respiratory Diseases, Dr. Edelman has published extensively in the field of pulmonary diseases and control of breathing. In 1990, he was named recipient of a MERIT award for the National Institutes of Health, National Heart, Lung and Blood Institute. He is the author of the *American Lung Association's Family Guide to Asthma and Allergies.*

A graduate of Brooklyn College, Dr. Edelman received his M.D. degree from New York University.

Dr. Edelman has appeared on a number of national news programs, including *Good Morning America, CBS Evening News, Dateline NBC* and *MSNBC.* He has been interviewed by several major newspapers and wire services, including *USA Today, Washington Post, Los Angeles Times, Reuters* and the *Associated Press.*

Who Is Celia Slom Vimont (writer)?

Celia Slom Vimont is a health and medical writer. A graduate of the Columbia School of Journalism, she has written for magazines, newspapers and wire services for both consumers and physicians. The former Director of Editorial Services for the American Lung Association, Celia served as in-house editor for books on asthma and smoking cessation for the association and continues to write about a variety of lung health issues. She is the writer of two previous books in the *Chicken Soup Healthy Living* series, *Weight Loss* and *Menopause*. Celia lives in New York City with her husband and son.

More Chicken Soup

Many of the stories in this book were submitted by readers just like you. If you would like more information on submitting a story, visit our Web site at *www.chickensoup.com*. If you do not have Web access, we can also be reached at:

Chicken Soup for the Soul®
PO Box 30880, Santa Barbara, CA 93130
Fax: 805-563-2945

Contributors

Vicki Armitage is the owner of Vicki's Dance Studios in central Louisiana and has been a guest on the Oprah Winfrey Show. Much change and time away from her roles have provided insight for her life's second journey and the memoir she will someday write. *vckilyn@aol.com*, 3215 Parkway Drive, Alexandria, LA 71301.

Emily Bamberger is 15 years old and lives with her mom, dad, her little sister, Elissa, and dog, Bindi, in Kansas City. Emily has had asthma for three years. She developed it at summer camp.

Jessica Berger is a college student from Missouri currently studying psychology. A published poet, featured in the 2005 edition of *Who's Who in Poetry*, this is Jessica's first short story to be published. Jessica's plans include authoring fiction and nonfiction.

Susanne Brent was born in Chicago and earned a journalism degree from Metro State College in Denver. Susanne now lives in Phoenix, Arizona, with her husband, Ed, and her sweet, old dog, Buddy. Recent publishing credits include nonfiction in *Cup of Comfort for Christmas* and *A Matter of Choice: 25 People Who Transformed Their Lives*.

Shari Davis Gonzales is the mother of two beautiful boys: Bradley, age nine, and Sydney, age five. She and her husband, Mike, have been married for 16 years and live in sunny Redington Beach, Florida. Shari has been an active volunteer with the American Lung Association for five years.

Renee Hall-Freeman is a choir director and public speaker. She resides in Columbus, Ohio, with her husband William and sons, Charles and Kevin, and daughter Kenee. Reneé can be contacted at *hallfreeman@aol.com*.

Jaye Lewis is an award-winning writer who believes that where there is breath there is hope. A severe asthmatic, Jaye looks for reasons to rejoice in the most difficult of circumstances. You can read more of Jaye's inspirational stories on her Web site at *www.entertainingangels.org*. E-mail Jaye at *jayelewis@comcast.net*.

Shawn Scott McSwain is a working mom who lives with her husband, Tom, and son, Jack, in Raleigh, North Carolina.

Felice Prager is a freelance writer from Scottsdale, Arizona, with credits in local, national and international publications. In addition to writing, she also works with adults and children with moderate to severe learning disabilities as a multisensory educational therapist.

Jessica Rogerson is 16 years old and lives in West Virginia with her mother, father, sister, two dogs and two cats. Jessica enjoys reading, listenning to music, playing piano, writing and drawing. She also enjoys being in 4-H. She plans to one day be a member of the FBI.

Joyce Stark lives in North East Scotland and works for the Community Mental Health. Her hobby is writing about people around her and those she meets on her travels in the United States. She has completed a series to introduce very young children to a second language and is currently working on a travel journal of her trips to "Small Town/Big City America." E-mail her at: *joric.stark@virgin.net.*

Anne Stopper is a freelance journalist and former Fulbright scholar to Ireland who lives and works between the United States and Ireland. Her articles have been published in newspapers from Washington, D.C., to northeastern Pennsylvania. She has also worked in broadcasting for National Public Radio's flagship news program *Morning Edition.*

Permissions

Also Available

Chicken Soup African American Soul
Chicken Soup Body and Soul
Chicken Soup Bride's Soul
Chicken Soup Caregiver's Soul
Chicken Soup Cat and Dog Lover's Soul
Chicken Soup Christian Family Soul
Chicken Soup Christian Soul
Chicken Soup College Soul
Chicken Soup Country Soul
Chicken Soup Couple's Soul
Chicken Soup Expectant Mother's Soul
Chicken Soup Father's Soul
Chicken Soup Fisherman's Soul
Chicken Soup Girlfriend's Soul
Chicken Soup Golden Soul
Chicken Soup Golfer's Soul, Vol. I, II
Chicken Soup Horse Lover's Soul
Chicken Soup Inspire a Woman's Soul
Chicken Soup Kid's Soul
Chicken Soup Mother's Soul, Vol. I, II
Chicken Soup Nature Lover's Soul
Chicken Soup Parent's Soul
Chicken Soup Pet Lover's Soul
Chicken Soup Preteen Soul, Vol. I, II
Chicken Soup Single's Soul
Chicken Soup Soul, Vol. I-VI
Chicken Soup at Work
Chicken Soup Sports Fan's Soul
Chicken Soup Teenage Soul, Vol. I-IV
Chicken Soup Woman's Soul, Vol. I, II
